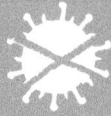

KEEP CALM
AND

WASH YOUR HANDS

DEAR PARENTS AND TEACHERS,

Congratulations on encouraging your children and students to become bilingual and bilingually literate!

It is a decision that will pay dividends to your child or student for many years to come! Research has shown that it is easier for children who learn a language before the age of 6 to adopt a native accent. Research also shows that bilingual children have increased cognitive capacities.

The goal of Young and Bilingual ™ is to accompany you and your children or students through the wonderful journey of becoming fully bilingual at a young age. The illustrations in each book are beautiful and colorful. Each book includes vocabulary words, a list of sight words used in the book, and phonic tips.

We have defined four different levels for our book series:

❶ Preschool-Kindergarten
Interactive reading, ideal for toddlers, who are discovering the world

❷ Preschool to Grade 1
Simple sentences ideal for pre-readers, who start learning how to read (under 125 words)

❸ Kindergarten to Grade 1
Short Story ideal for beginner autonomous readers (under 250 words)

❹ Kindergarten to Grade 2
Short Story, which includes life lessons and cultural discoveries (under 500 words)

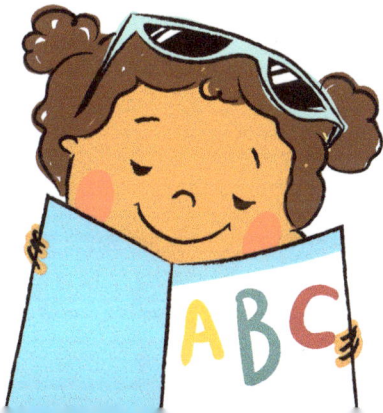

Young and Bilingual ™ offers FREE supporting bilingual material on its website www.lapetitepetra.com to assist you and your children and students on this great journey of bilingualism. We welcome your feedback to improve continuously. Stay in touch with us, and, most importantly, enjoy the journey!

DEDICATION

This book is dedicated to the families all over the world who suffered directly or indirectly from the Coronavirus. May we find meaning in this experience and come out stronger, more resilient than ever.

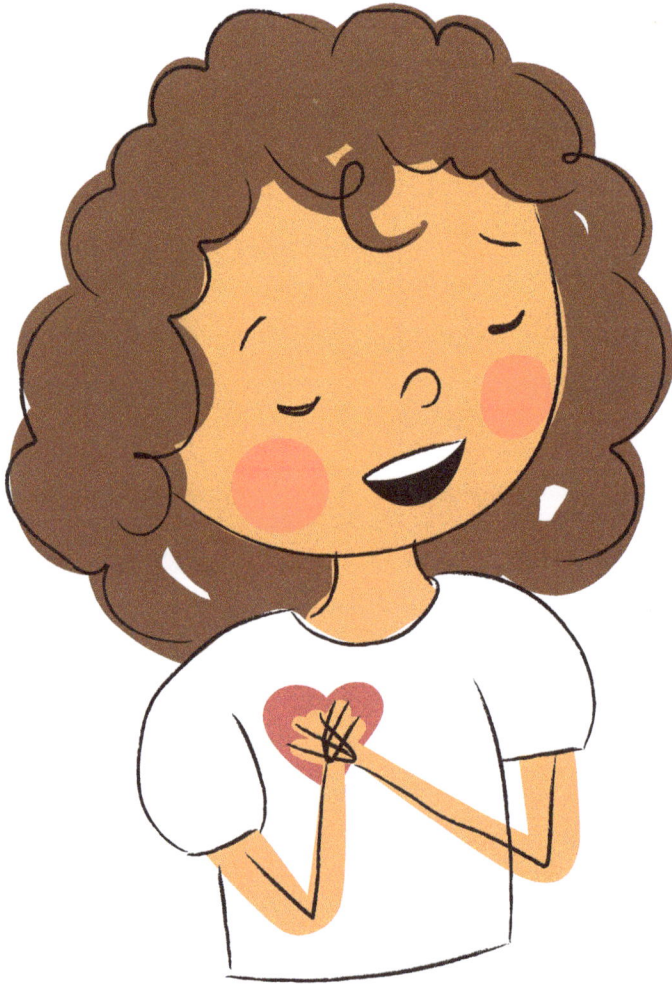

SPECIAL THANKS

To all the heroes around the world who put their life at risk to protect the victims of COVID-19. The world is a better place because of you.

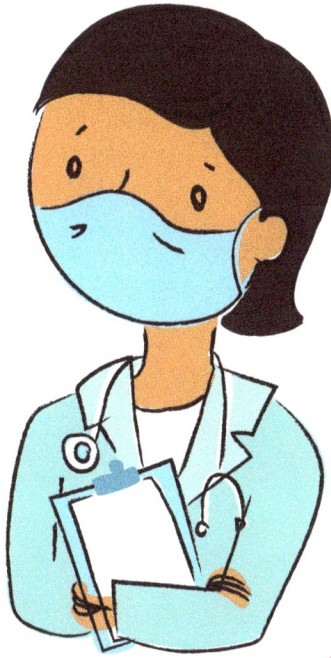

Publisher's Cataloging-In-Publication Data
(Prepared by Xponential Learning, Inc.)
Names: Kanzki, Krystel Armand, author. I Vynokurova, Oksana, illustrator.
Title: La Petite Pétra. The Coronavirus Explained for kids / Krystel Armand Kanzki ; illustrated by Oksana
Vynokurova.
Other Titles: The Coronavirus Explained for kids
Description: [Miami, Florida] : Xponential Learning Inc, 2020. I Series:
La Petite Pétra. English. I Interest age level: 005-010. I Summary: 'Petra and Lili explain to kids what the
Coronavirus is and how it gets transmitted from one person to the next. They show children what to do to
protect themselves from catching and spreading the virus'--Provided by publisher.

Identifiers: ISBN 9781949368291

ISBN: 978-1-949368-29-1

First Publication: March 2020
XPONENTIAL LEARNING INC

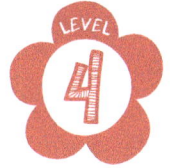

La Petite Pétra™

THE CORONAVIRUS
EXPLAINED FOR KIDS

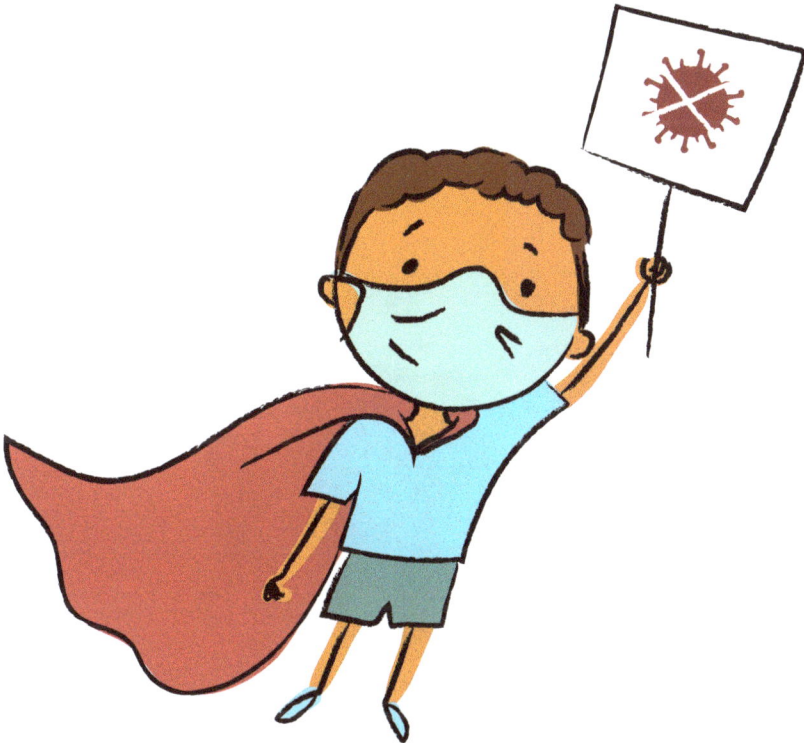

LEVEL 4

Krystel Armand Kanzki

Illustrated by Oksana Vynokurova

Everyone is talking about the coronavirus. What is it?

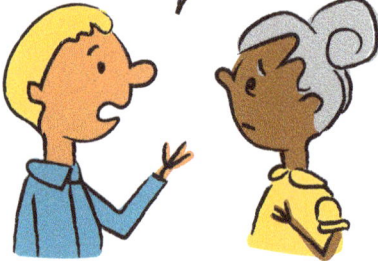

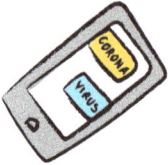

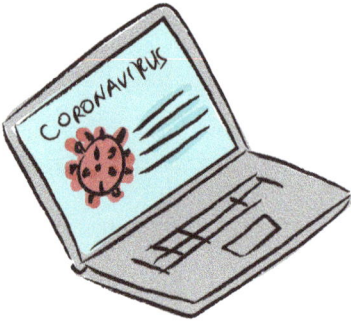

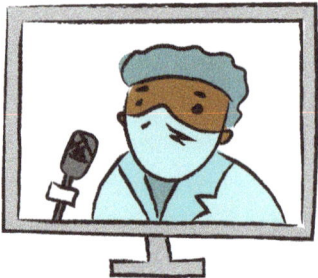

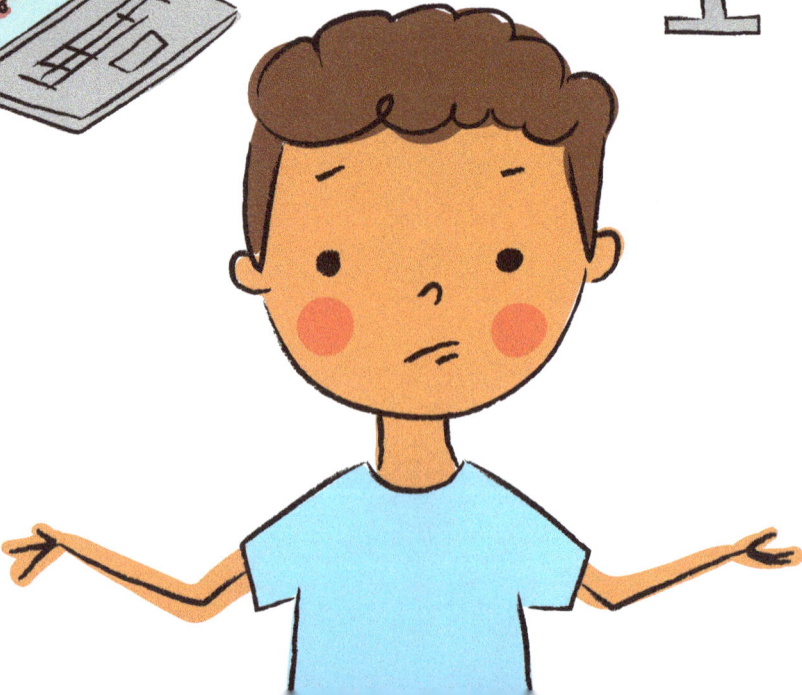

Under a microscope the virus looks like a solar crown.

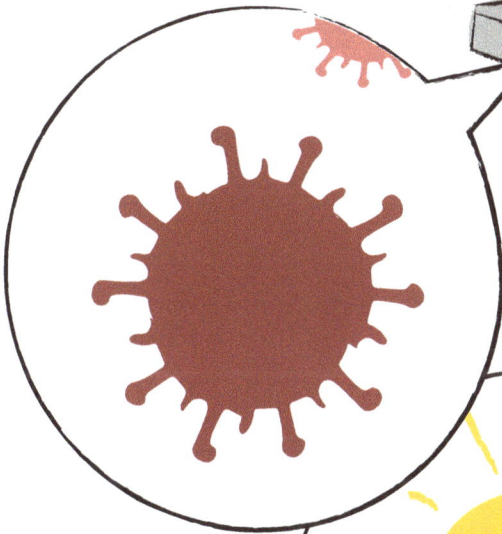

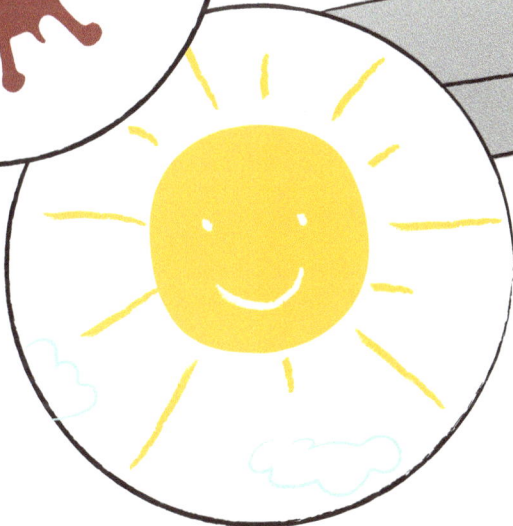

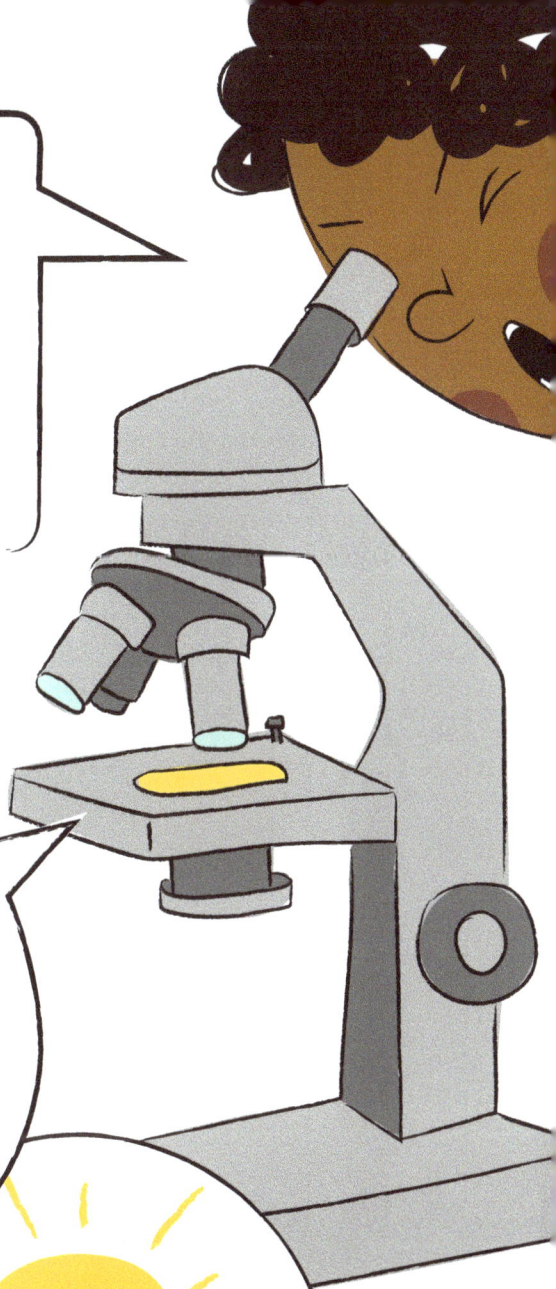

It is a virus that causes a disease called COVID-19.

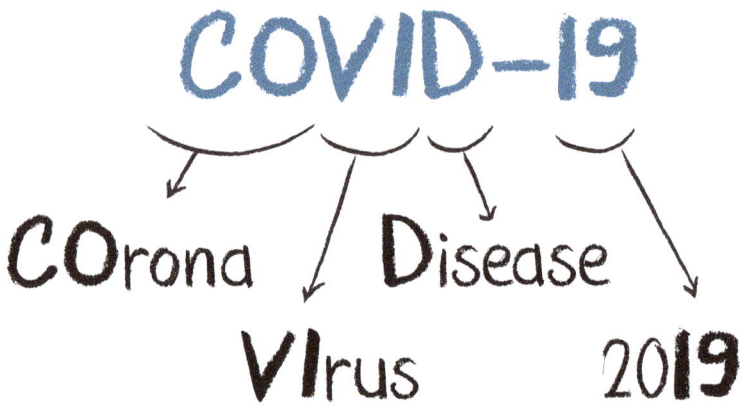

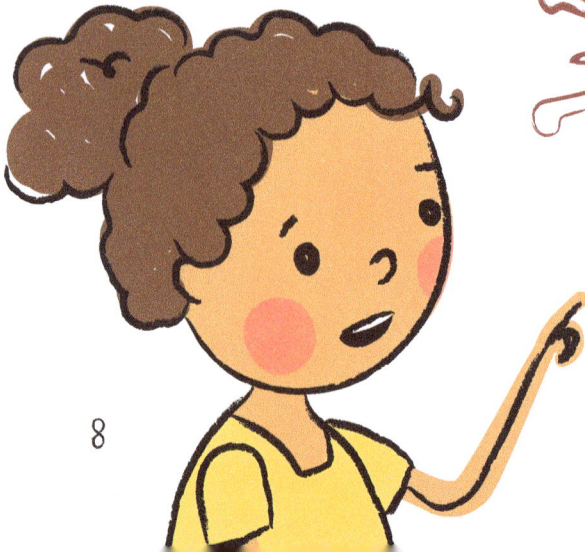

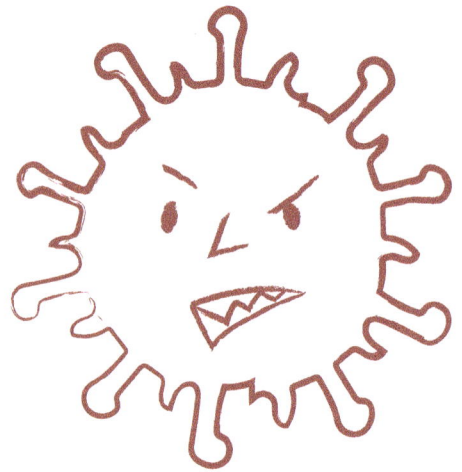

COVID-19

COrona Disease
VIrus 2019

It has made a lot of people sick all around the world.

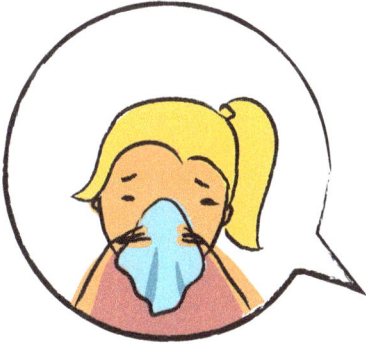

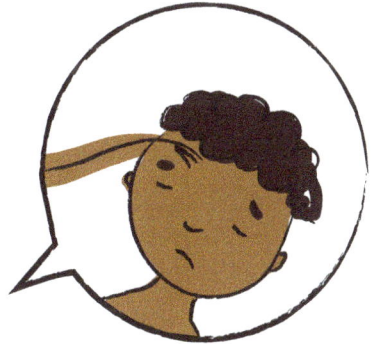

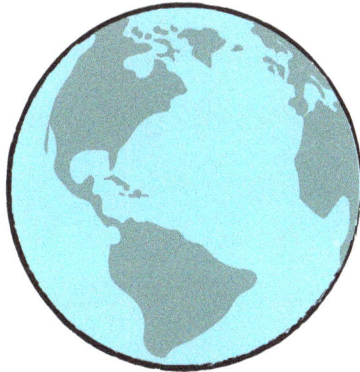

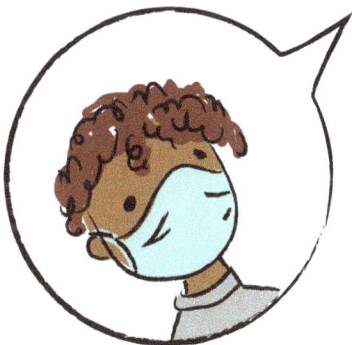

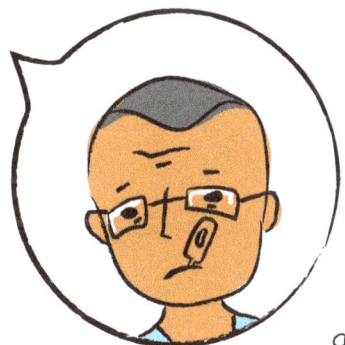

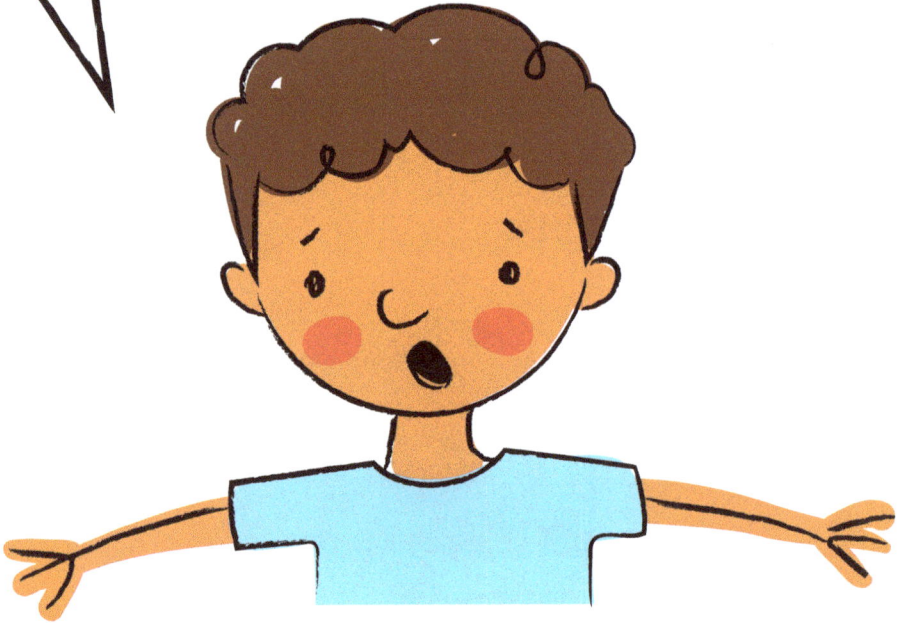

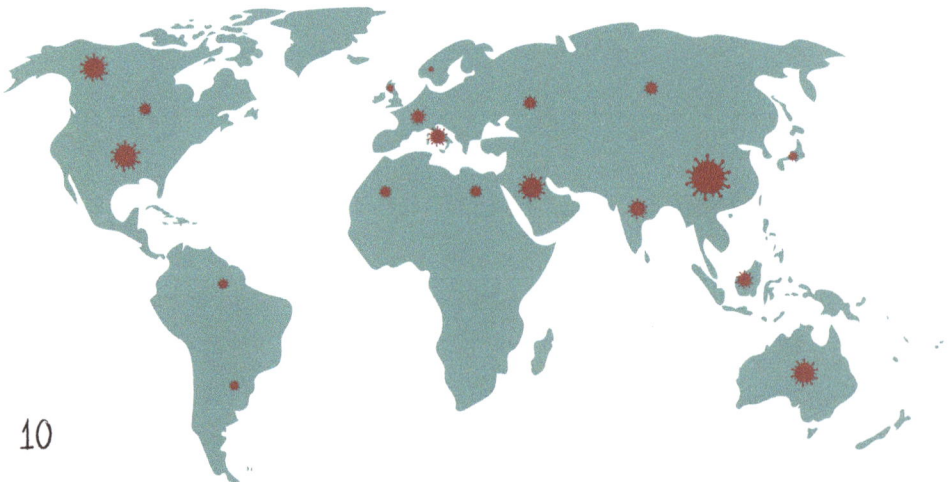

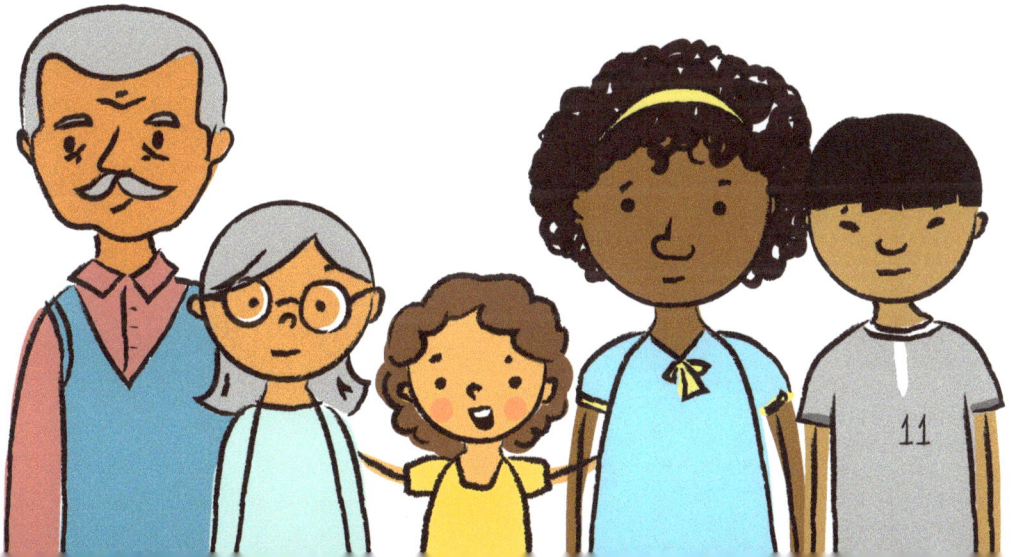

Yes, it does not matter what you look like, how old you are, what your skin color is, where you come from or what language you speak, you can get sick.

How is the virus transmitted from one person to another?

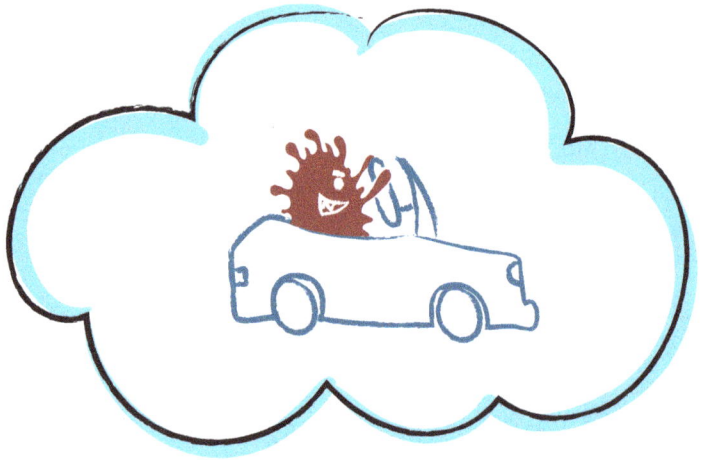

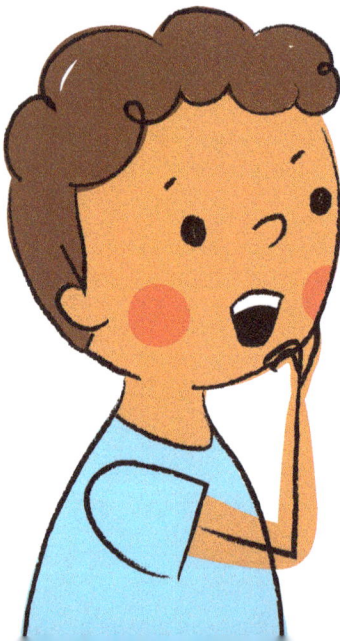

When a person who has caught the COVID-19 coughs, sneezes, talks, or even exhales close to other people, he can get these people sick.

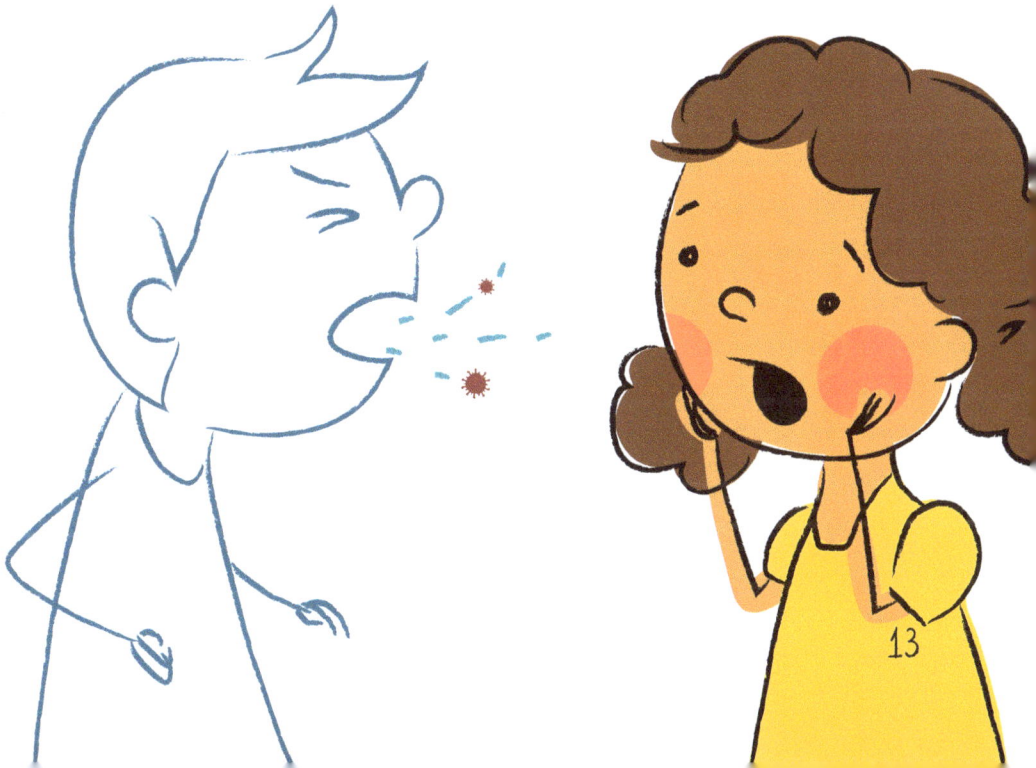

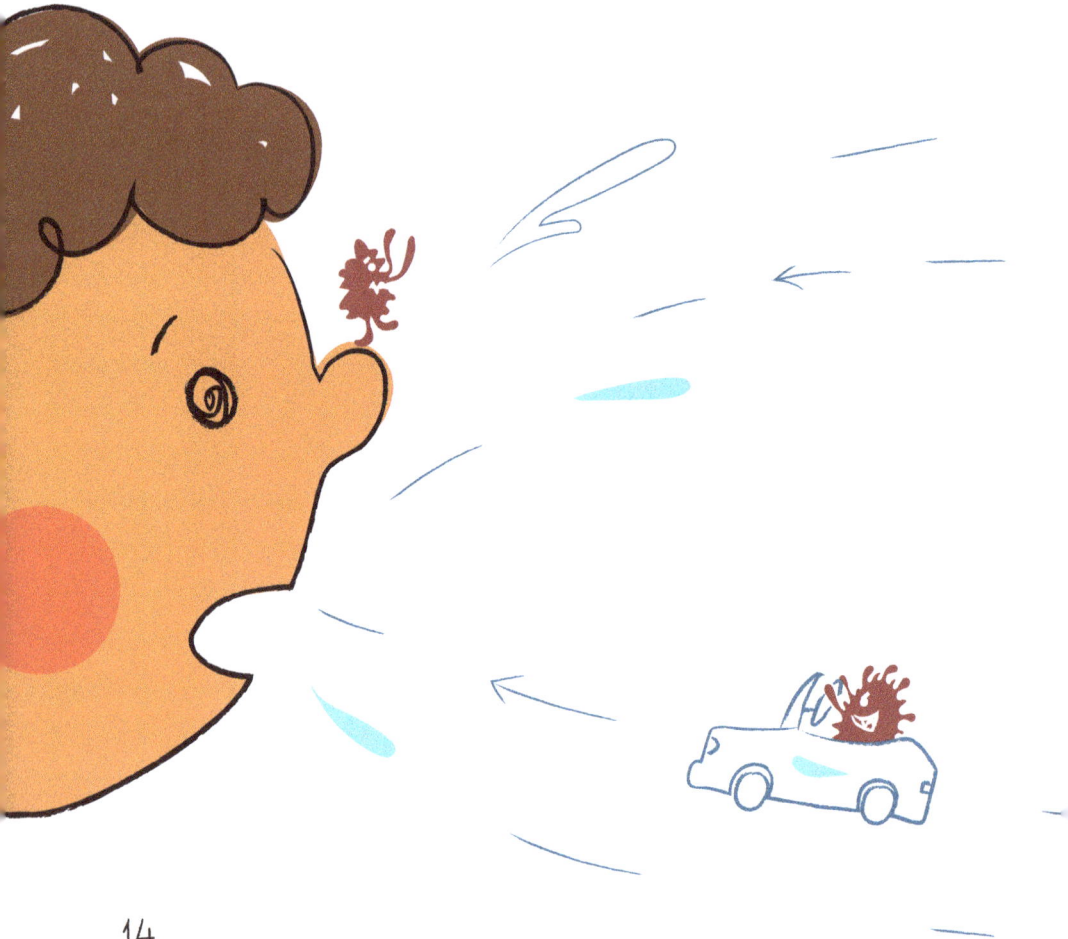

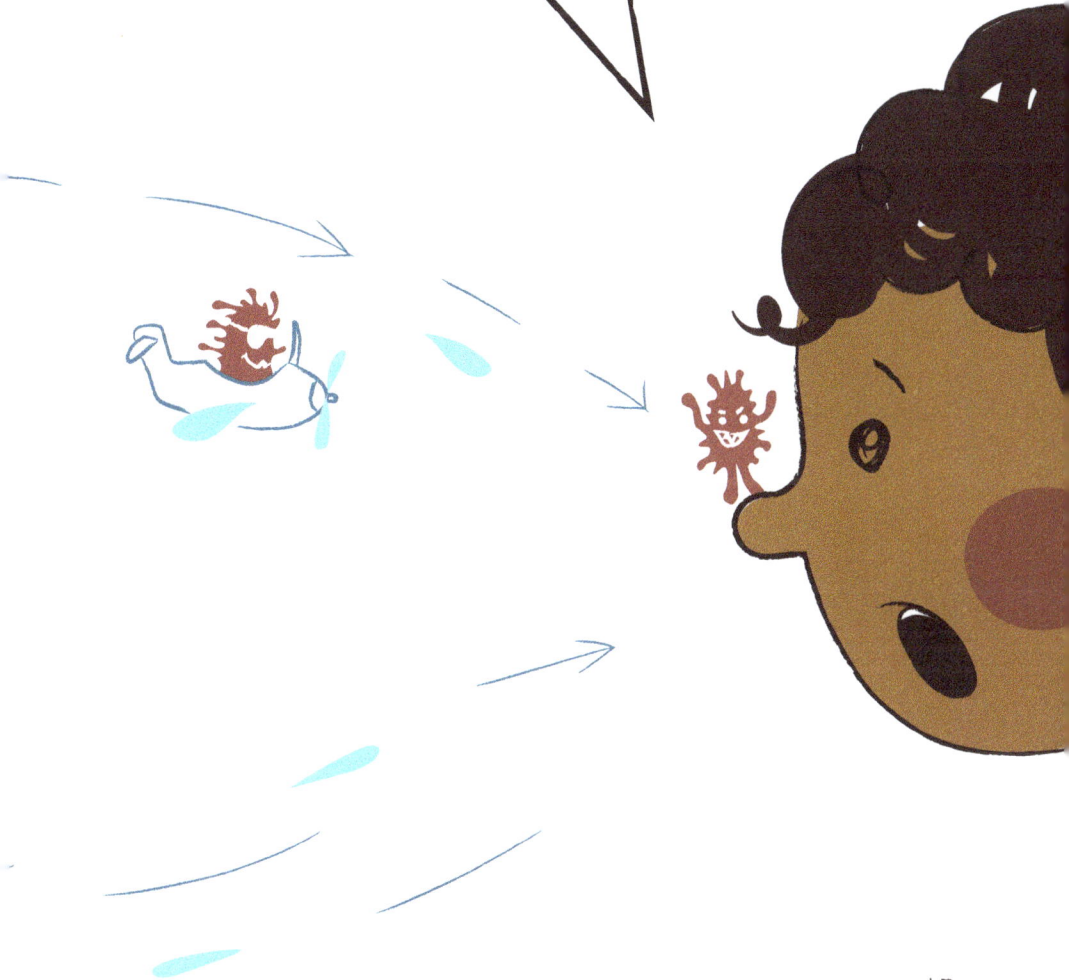

If the little drops produced from his nose or mouth land in the mouth or nose of people nearby, then they can get sick.

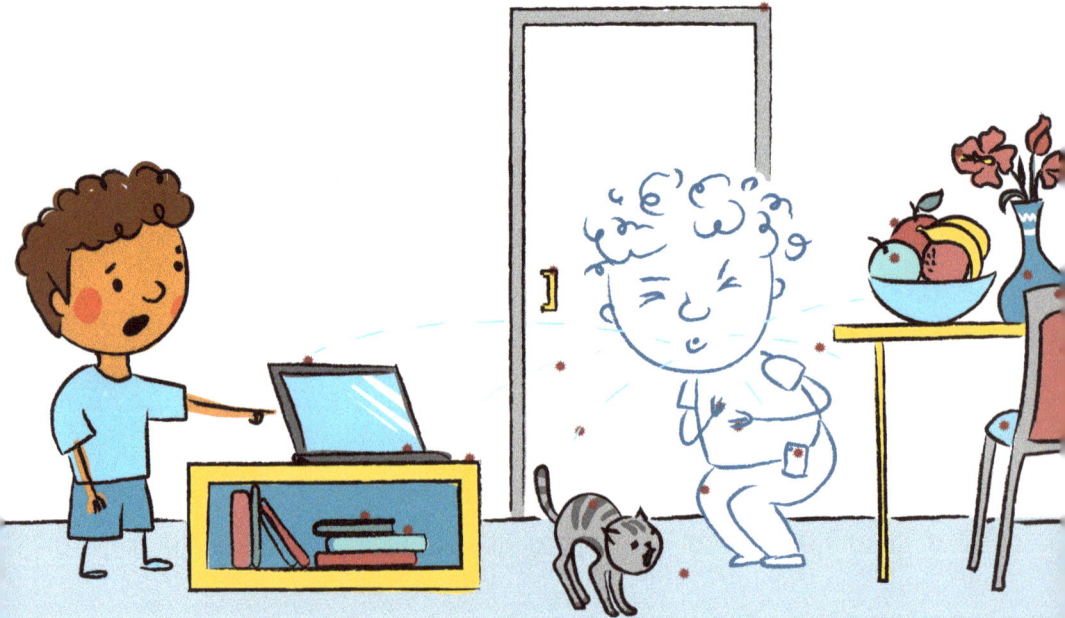

How about if the droplet lands on our hand or on an object, like a table, a book, or a phone?

KIDS,
FIND HOW MANY THINGS WILL GET INFECTED.

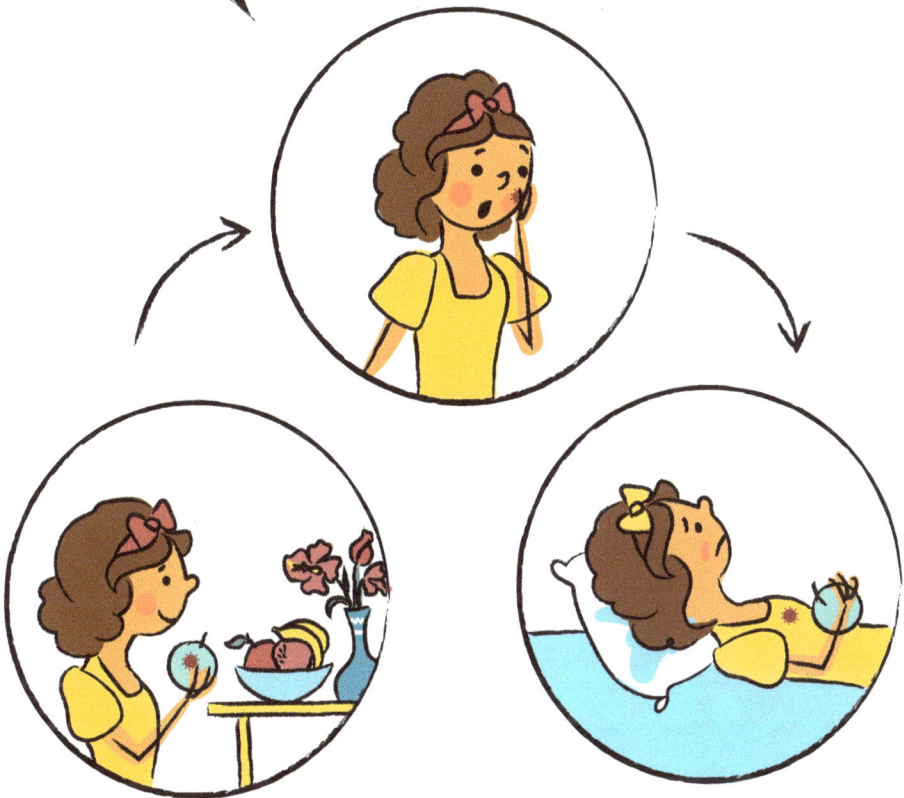

Great question! If a droplet lands on an object, and you touch that object, then you touch your eyes, mouth or nose with that infected hand, you can get sick too!

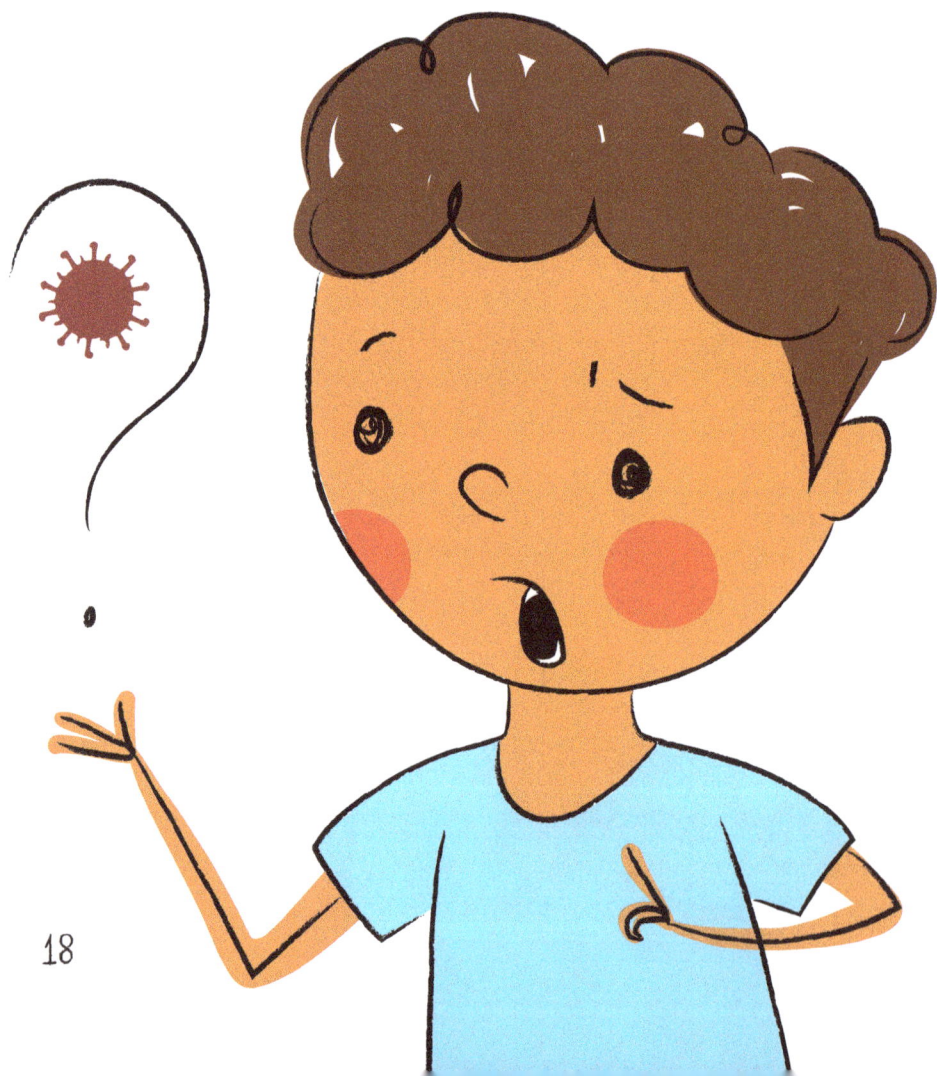

The symptoms are similar to the flu:

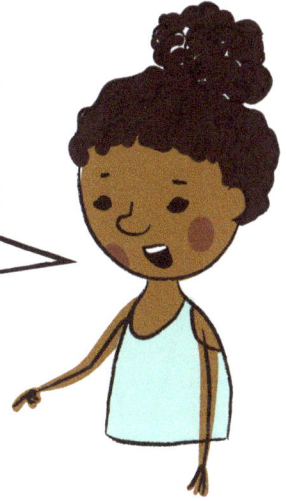

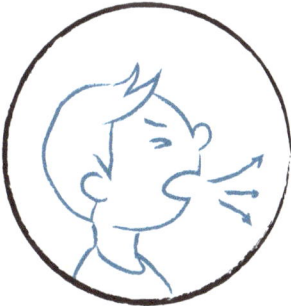

Dry itchy cough

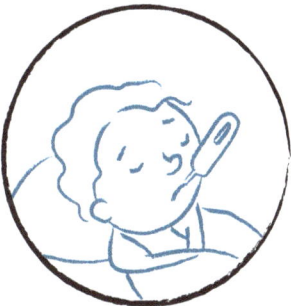

Fever

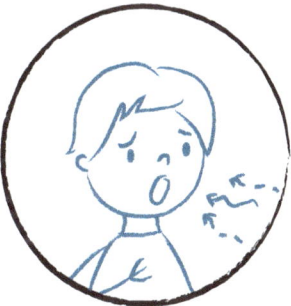

Difficulty breathing

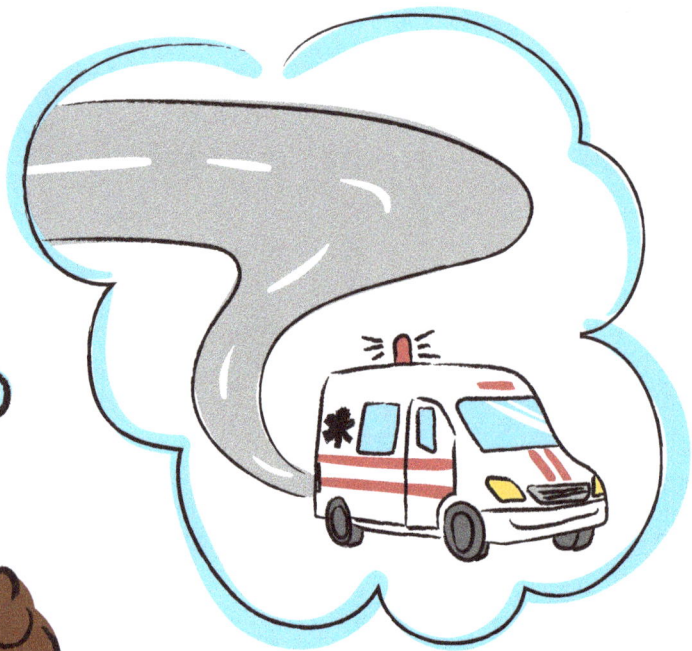

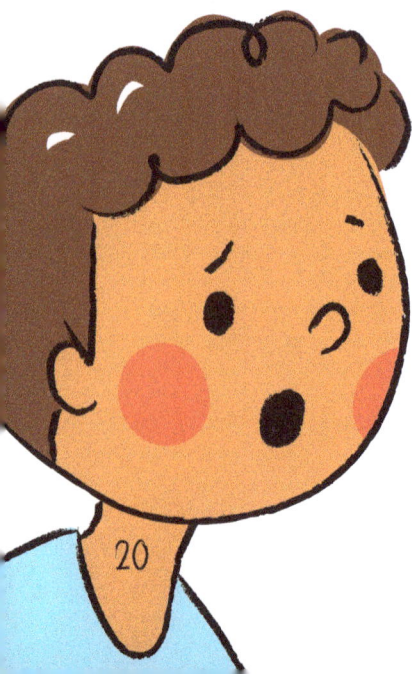

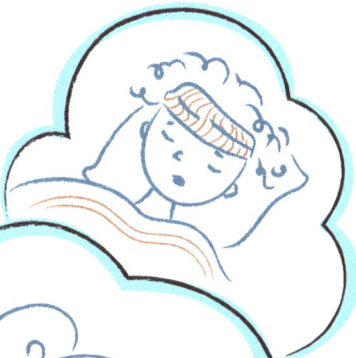

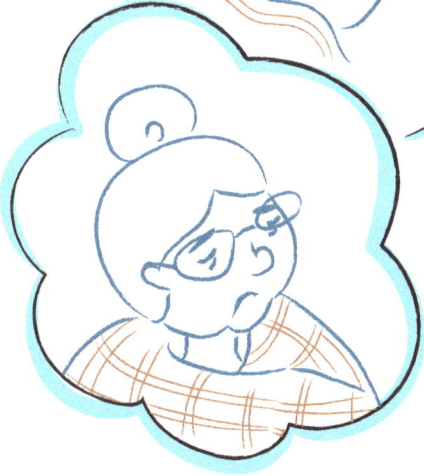

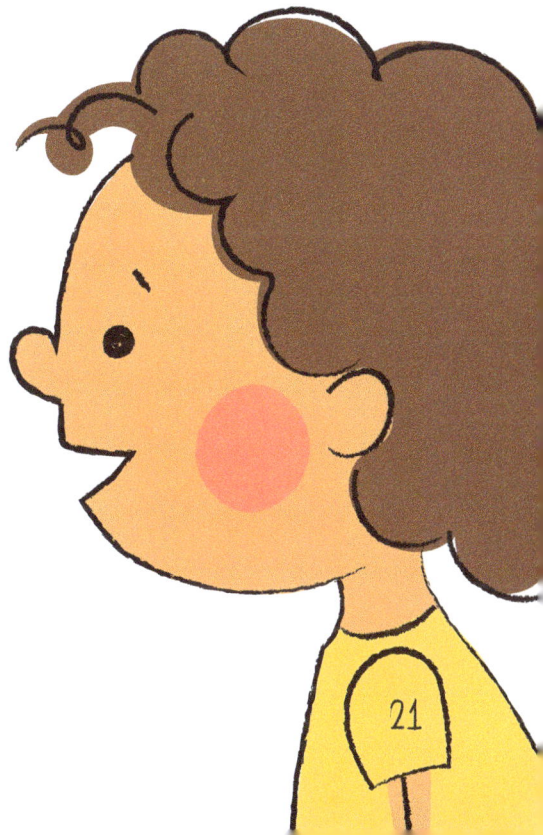

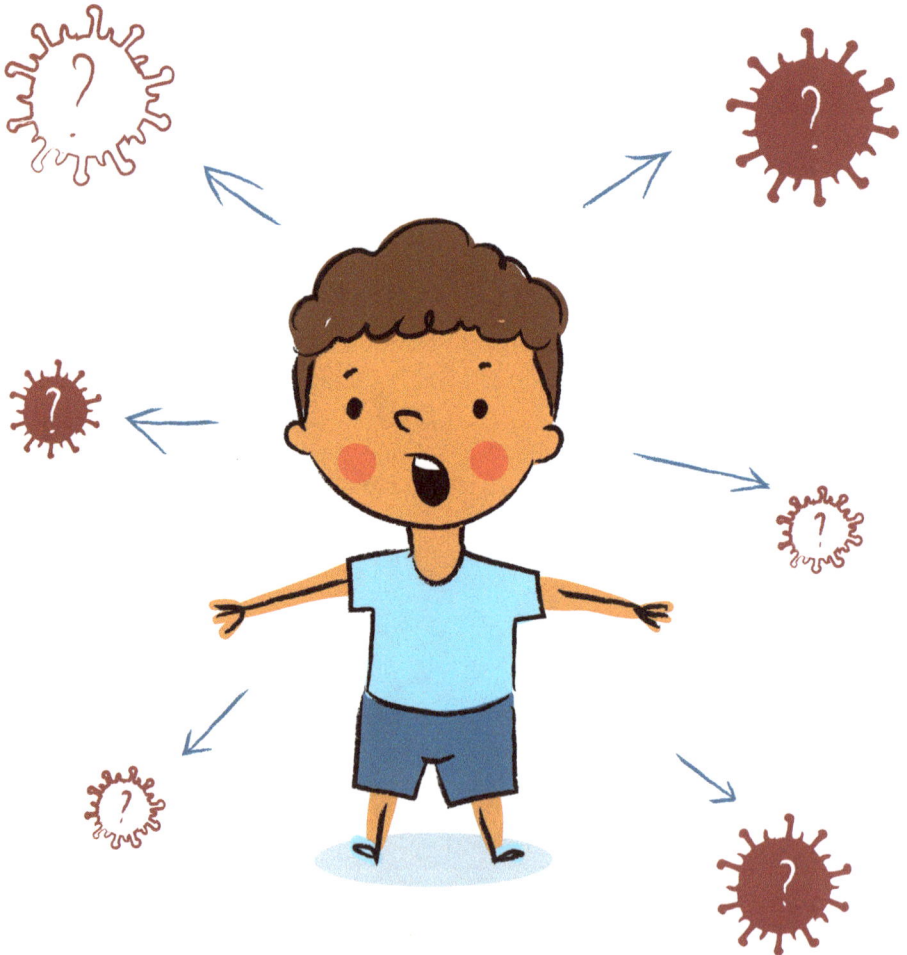

Can someone who does not get sick from the virus make someone else very sick?

Yes, especially since you can be a carrier of COVID-19 even if you don't know you are a carrier.

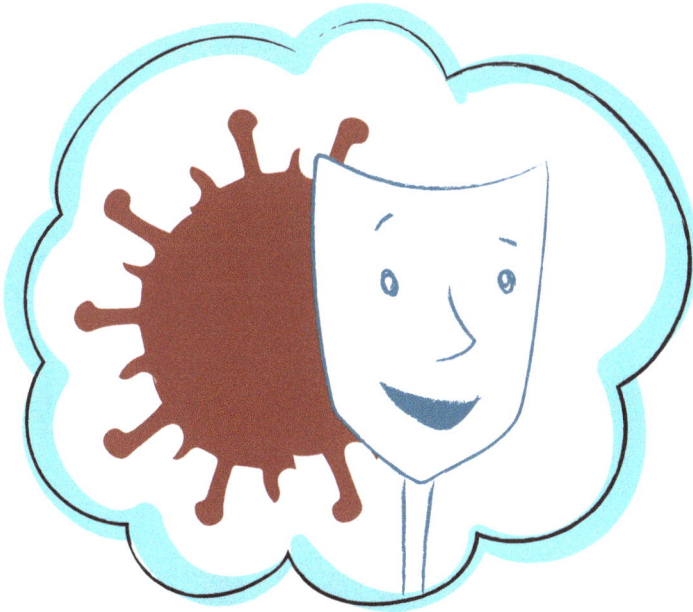

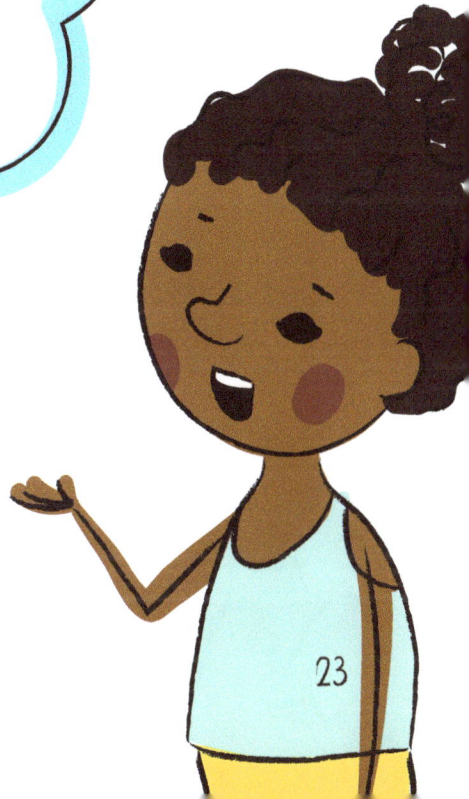

23

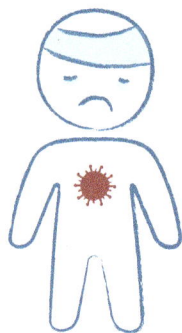

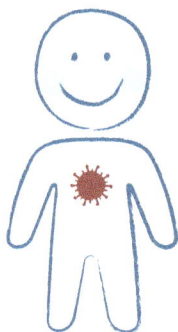

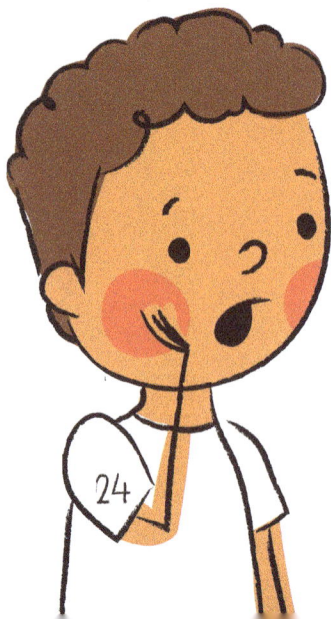

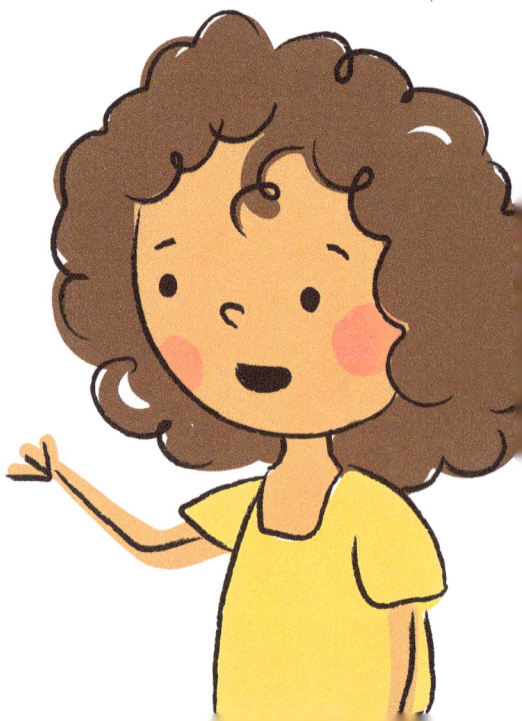

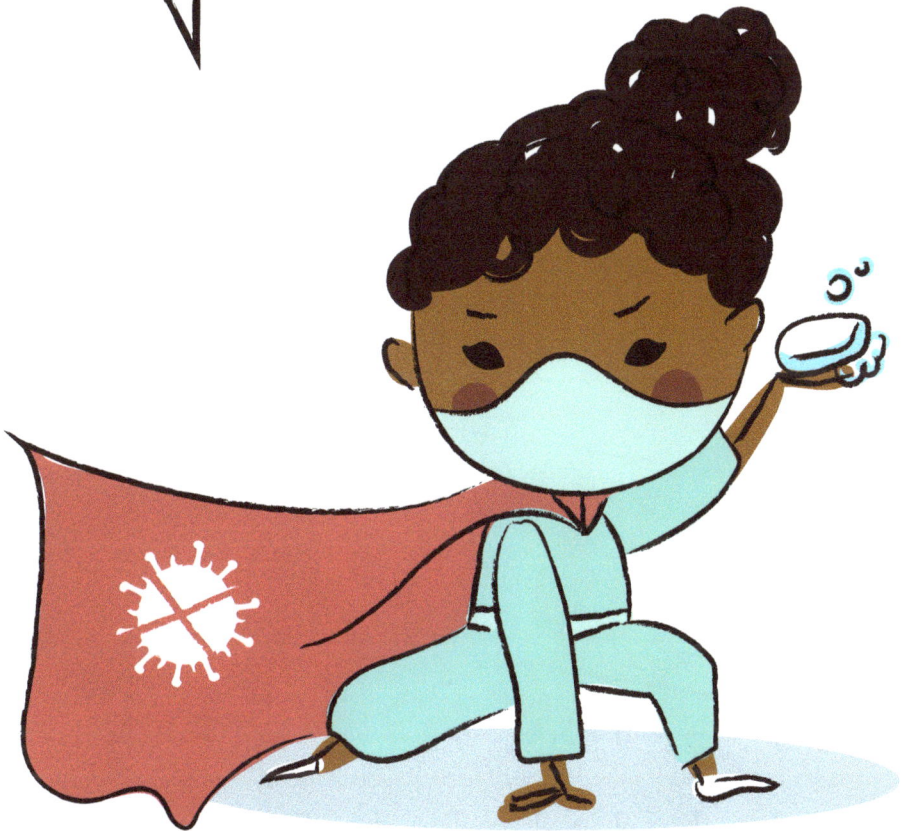

25

1 WASH YOUR HANDS WITH SOAP

ⓐ Make a lot of suds with the soap

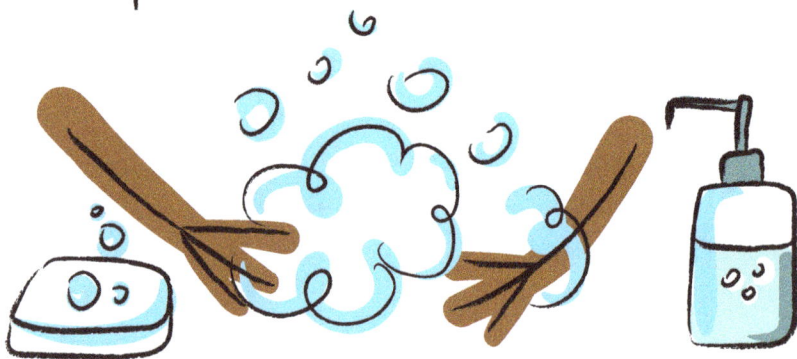

ⓑ Wash your hands for at least 20 seconds

Happy Birthday to you,
Happy Birthday to you,
Happy Birthday dear,
Happy Birthday to you!

× 3

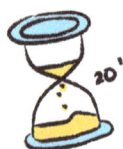

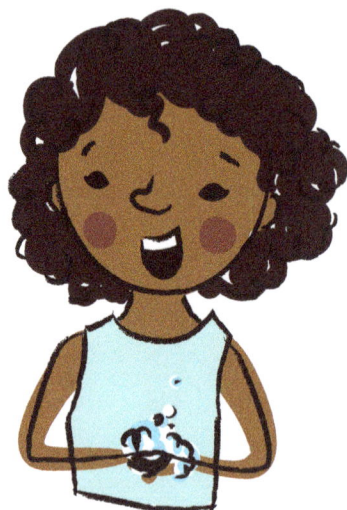

c Wash the hands after using the bathroom or being in public places (playgrounds, stores, buses)

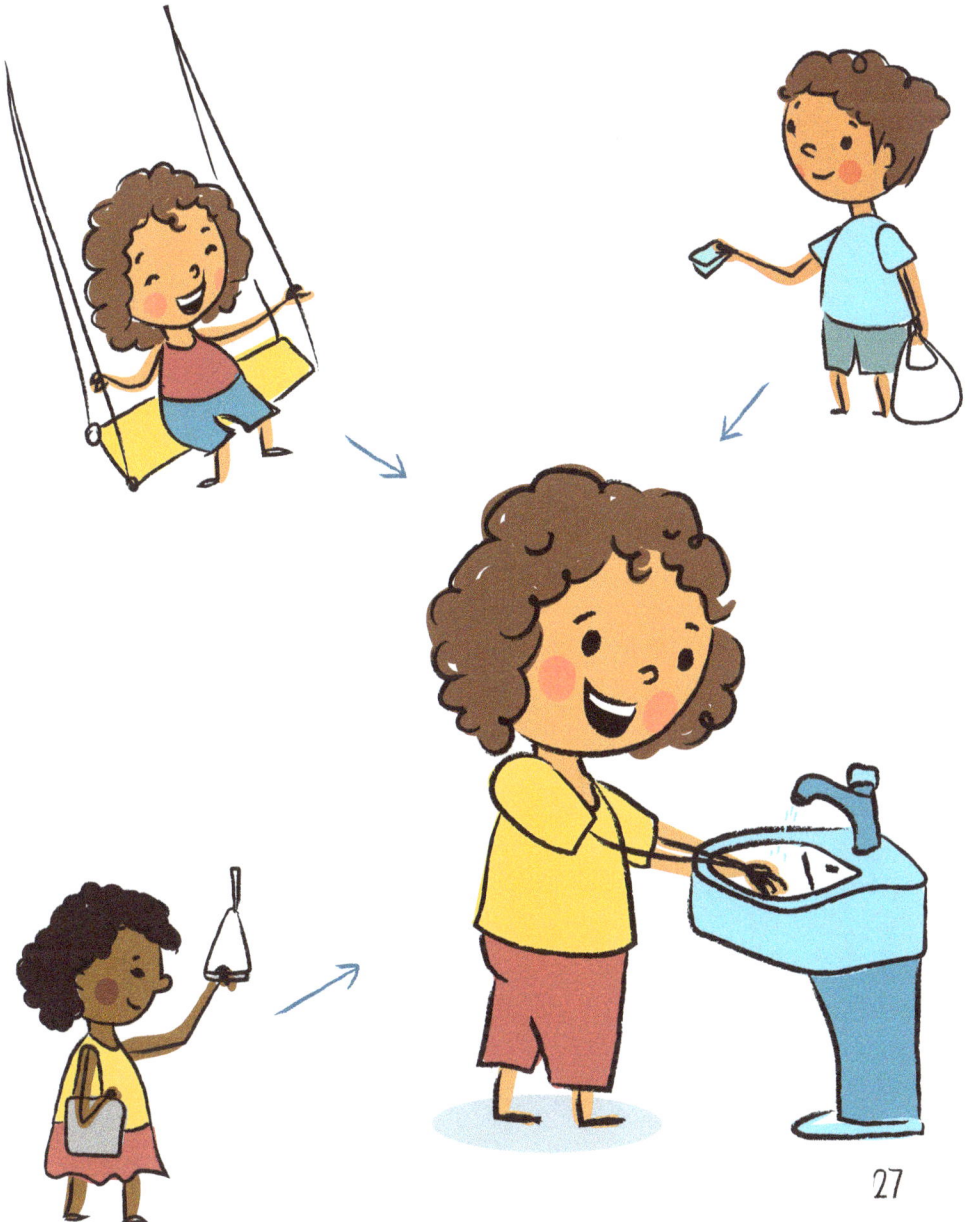

2 SNEEZE IN YOUR ELBOW

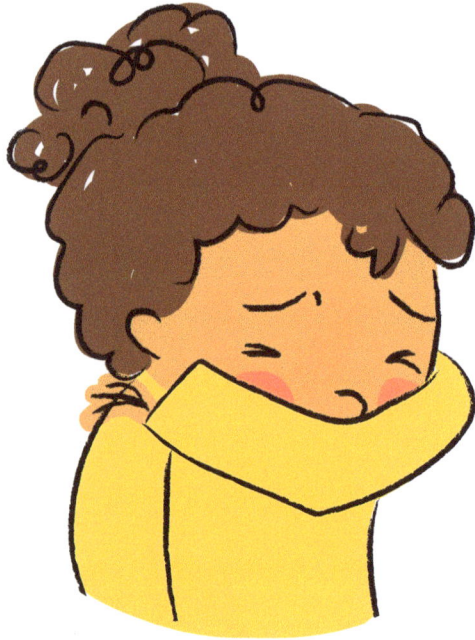

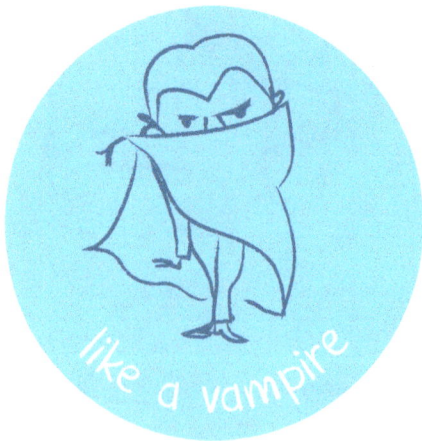

like a vampire

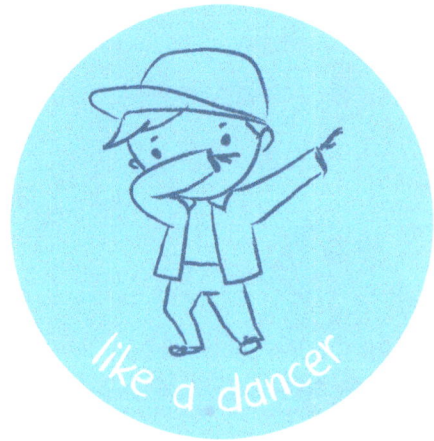

like a dancer

AVOID TOUCHING YOUR EYES, MOUTH, AND NOSE!

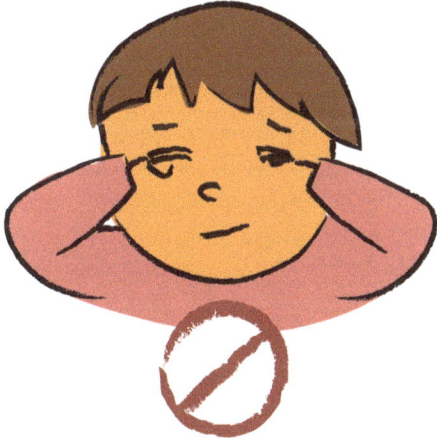

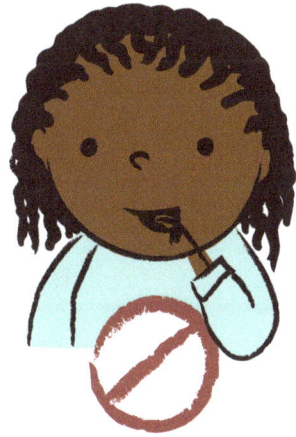

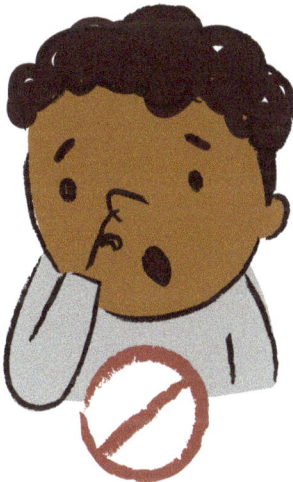

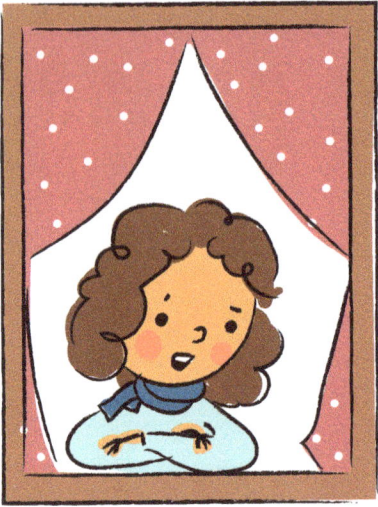

You need to stay at home as much as possible, ESPECIALLY IF YOU ARE SICK.

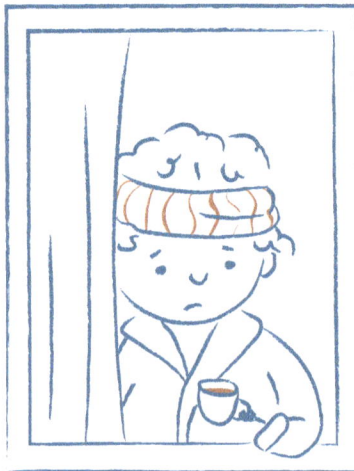

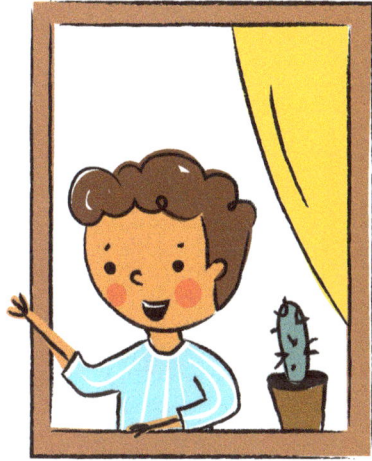

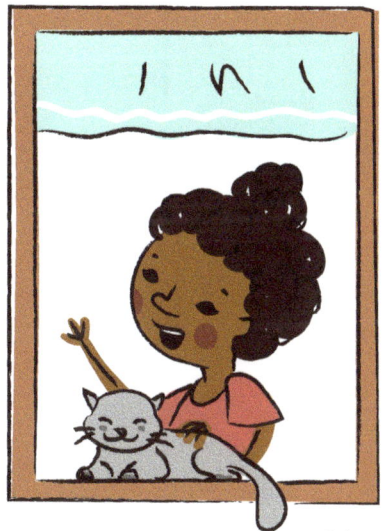

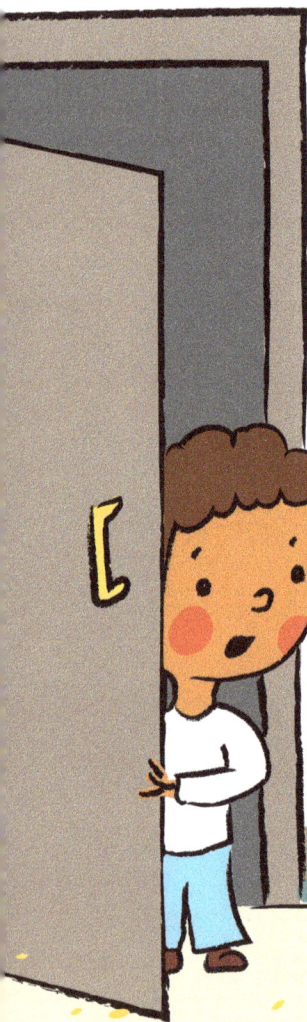

What to do if
I need go out?

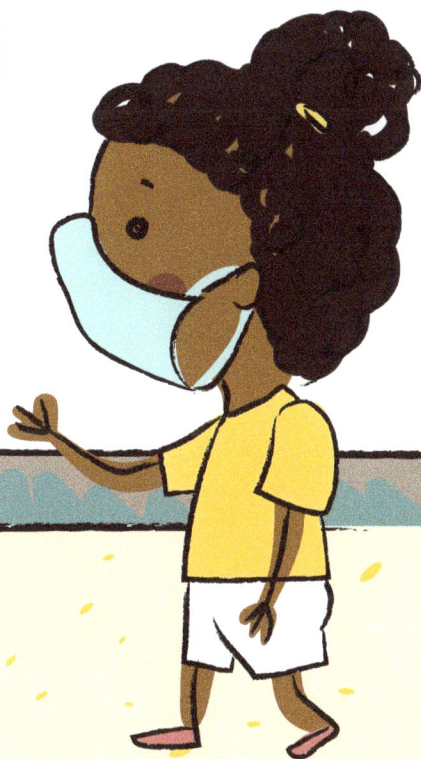

If you go out, you have to wear a mask and practice social distancing: stay far from others!

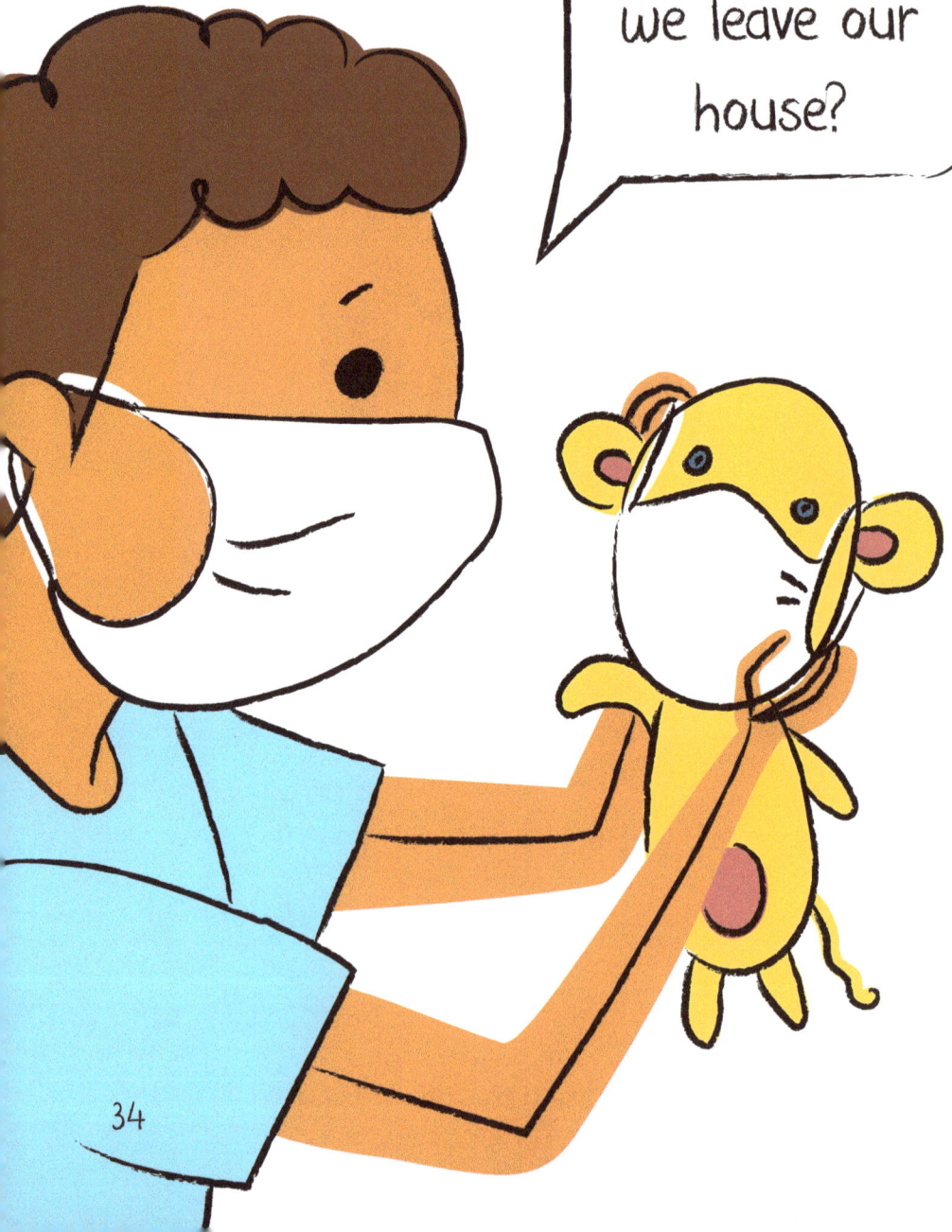

Why do we have to wear a mask when we leave our house?

Most potentially infected droplets can be caught by a mask. When we all wear a mask, we all protect one another.

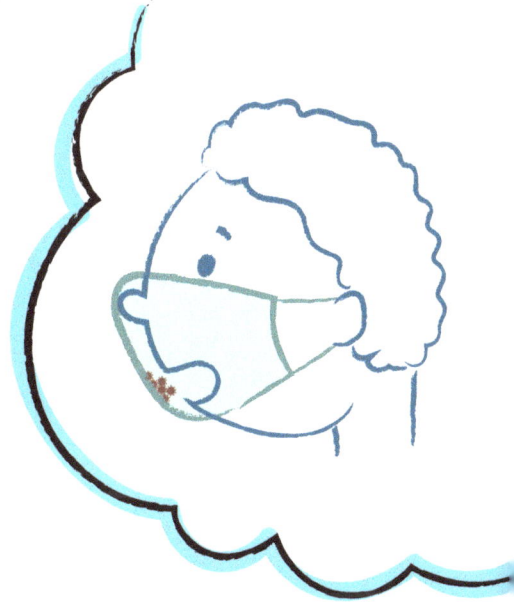

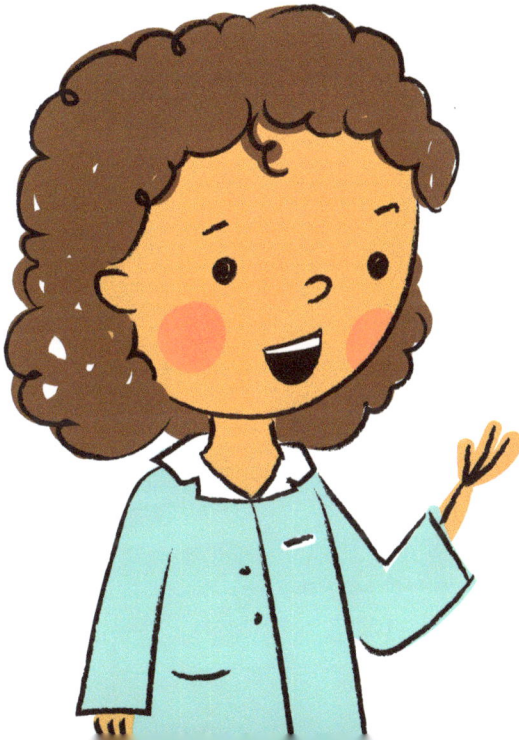

COVID-19 carrier*	Healthy person	Protection level

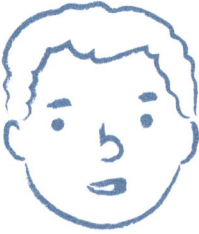 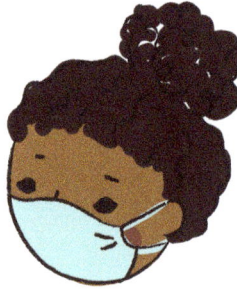 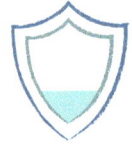

least

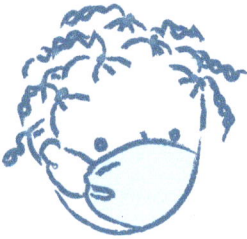 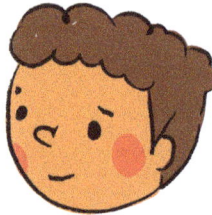 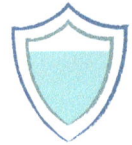

some

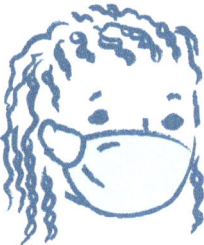 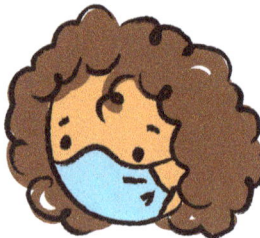 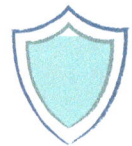

maximum

* this person may be symptom free

WEAR A MASK!

Even if you don't know you are carrier of COVID-19, you will not spread the disease.

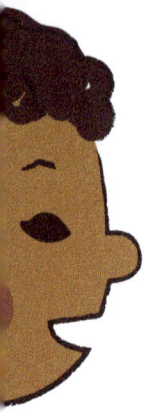

You can create a reusable mask yourself.
The most important thing is to cover your nose and mouth.

1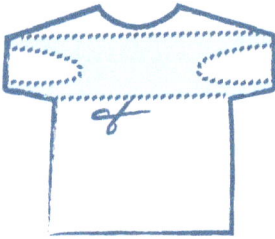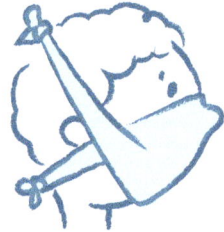

2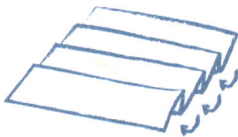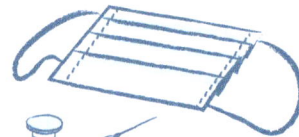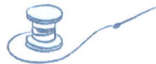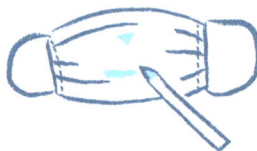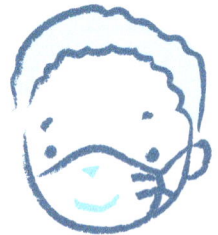

3

 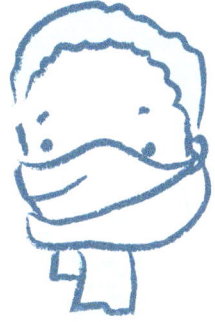

4

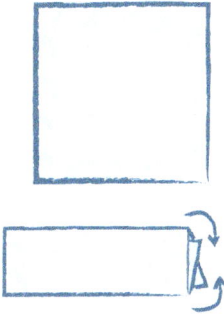 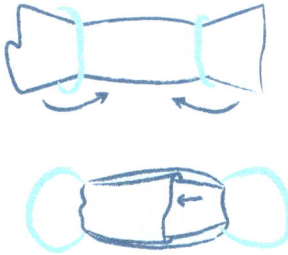 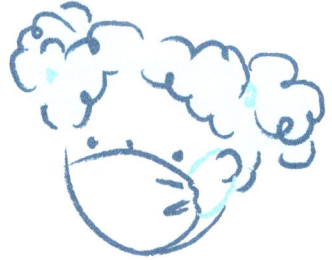

 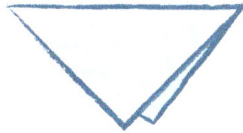 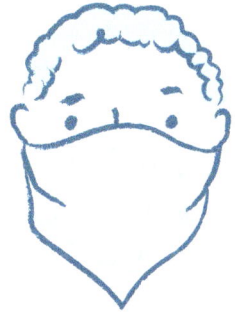

5

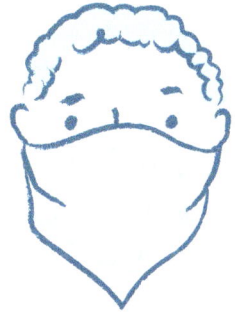

> **!** It's important to change mask every 2-3 hours and wash or iron after each usage.

We have to practice social distancing.

What is that?

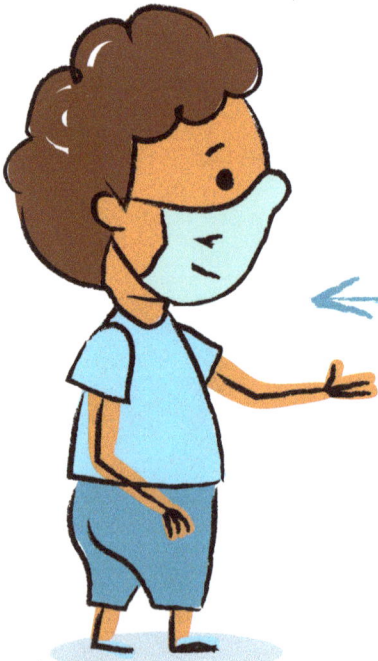

6 ft / 2 m

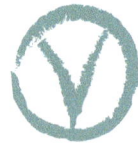

It's keeping a distance of at least 6 feet between us and other people so that droplets of an infected person cannot reach us.

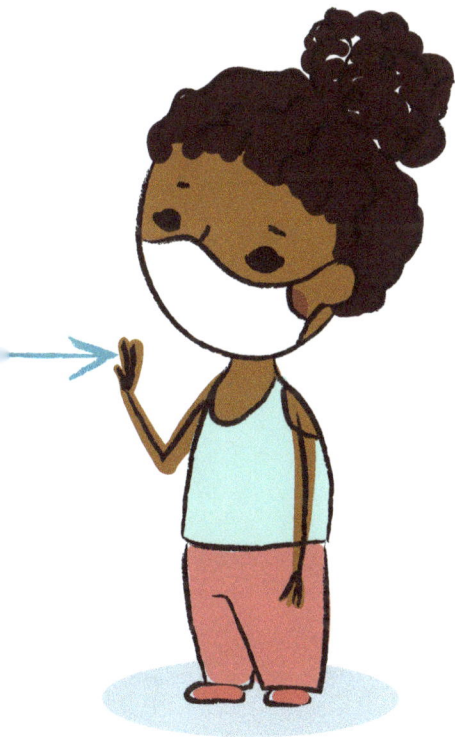

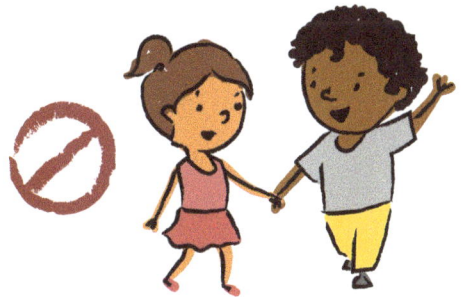

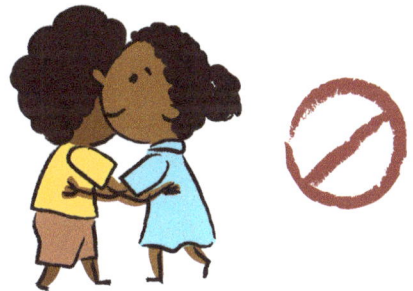

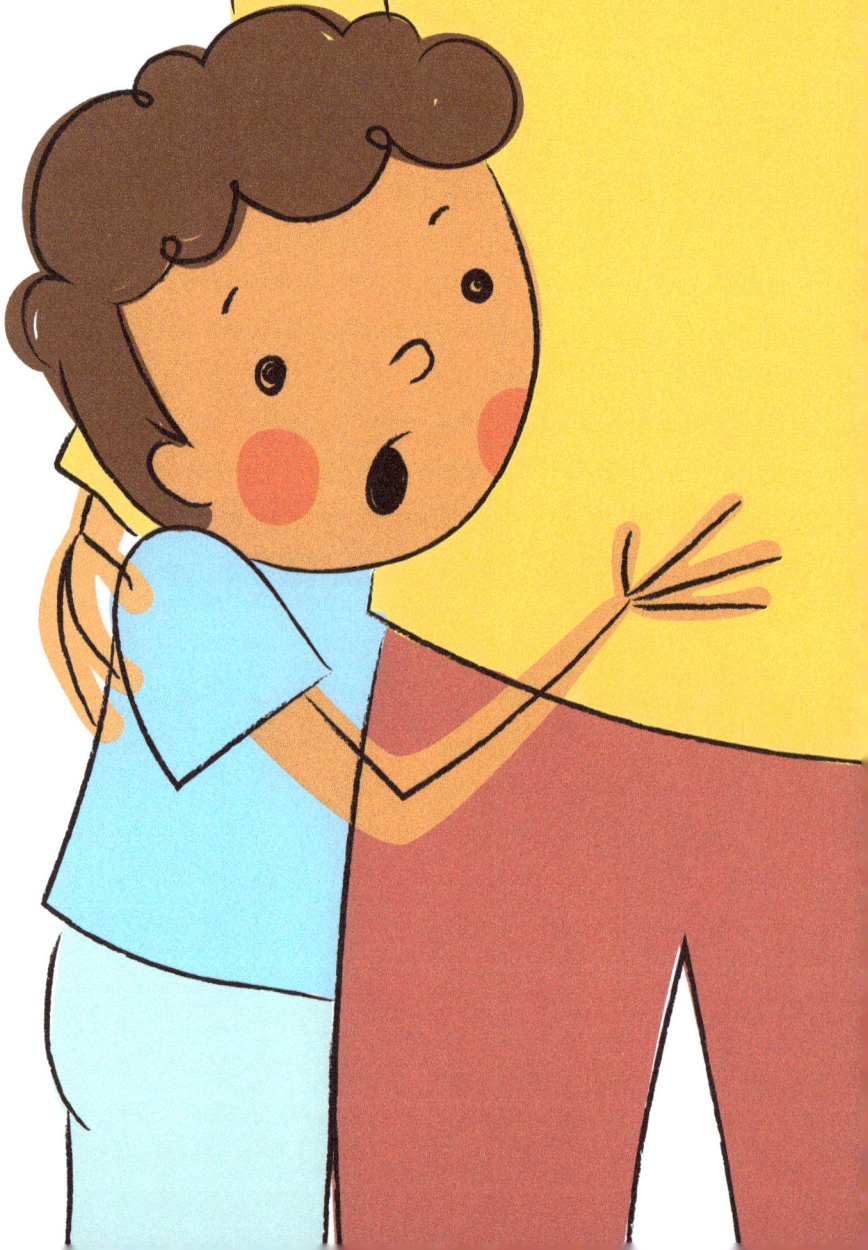

Should I worry?

There are a lot of people all around the world who are working hard to protect you.

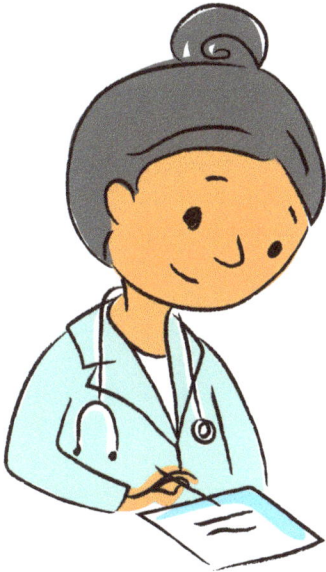

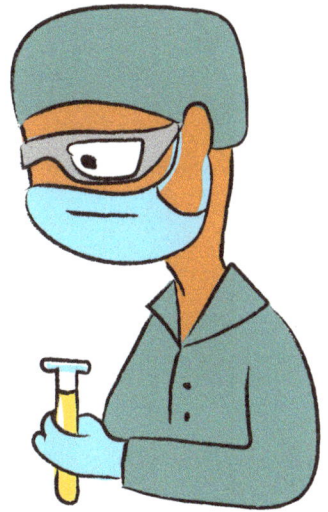

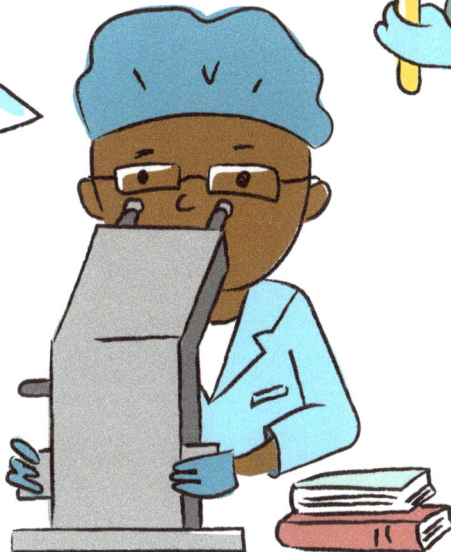

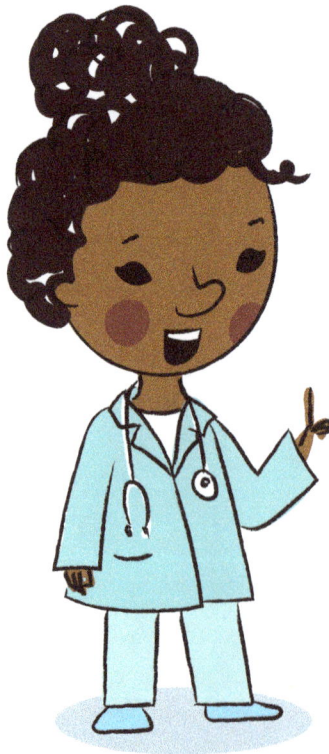

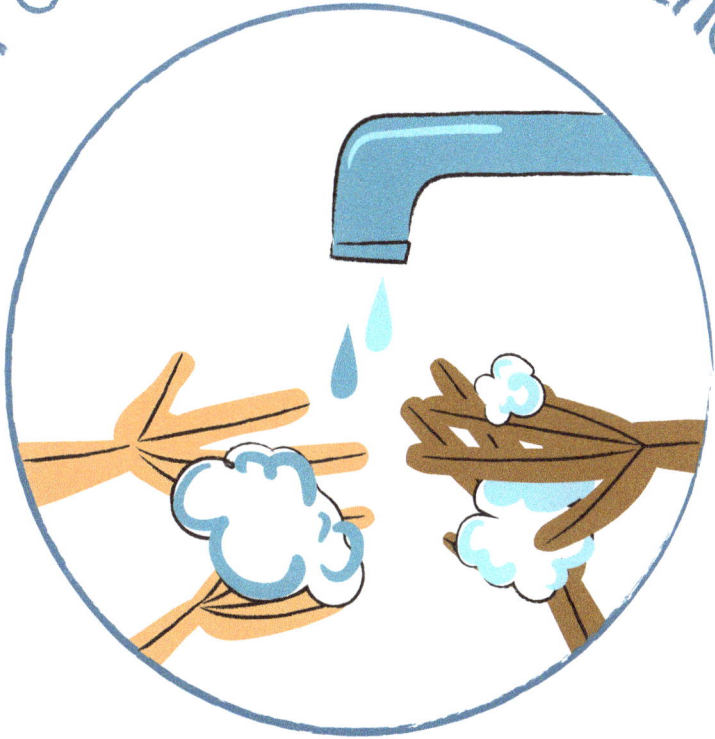

You can make a difference!

See you all soon!

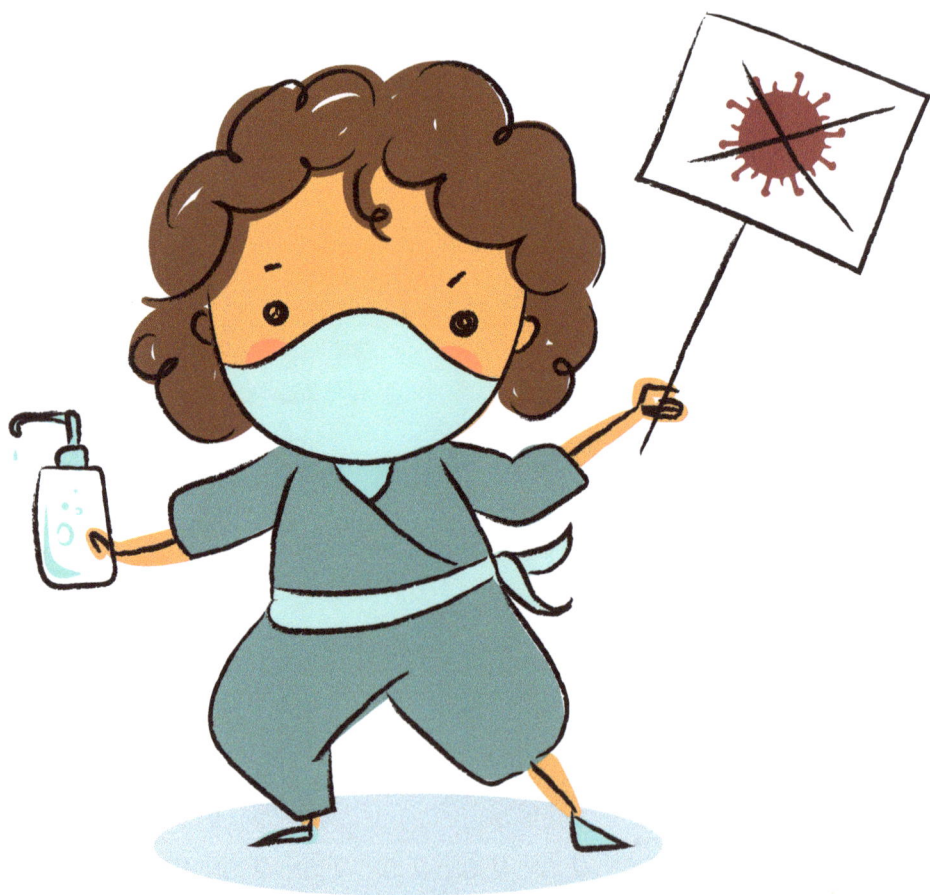

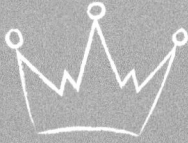

crown

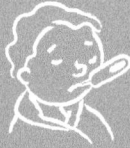

sick

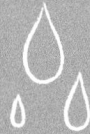

droplets

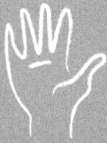

hand

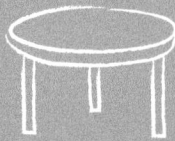

table

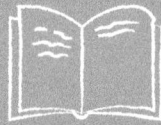

book

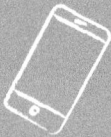

phone

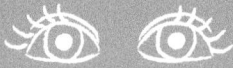

eyes

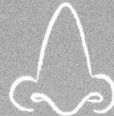

nose

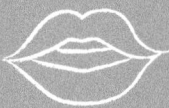

mouth

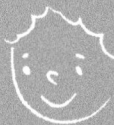

face

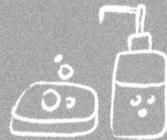

soap

YOUNG & BILINGUAL SIGHT WORDS TIPS

Sight words are words that don't follow the rules of spelling or syllable decoding. Children are taught as pre-readers to memorize sight words as a whole, by sight, so that they can recognize them immediately (within a few seconds). The goal is to read sight words without having to use decoding skills.

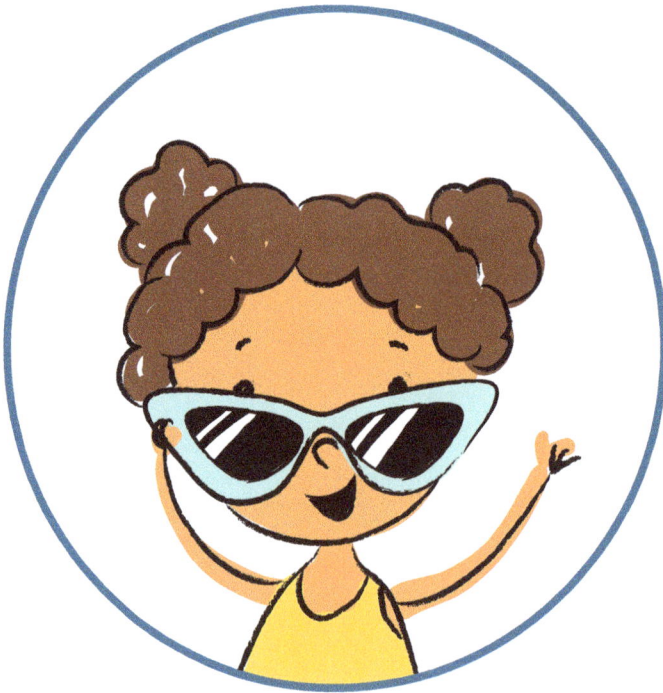

SIGHT WORDS FROM THE BOOK

position

in on

action

has do
can will be have

pronouns

you your

our it we

basic

the what is a that
of all from not or and
one an are to who with but
no very why at by

SHORT VOWELS VS. LONG VOWELS

- 'Long vowel' is the term used to refer to vowel sounds whose pronunciation is the same as its letter name. The five vowels of the English language are 'a', 'e', 'i', 'o', 'u'.
- Each letter has a corresponding short vowel sound.
- When a word has two vowels, usually, the first vowel is pronounced as a long vowel and the second vowel is silent.
- The vowel 'i' and 'o' have the long vowel sound when followed by two or more consonants.

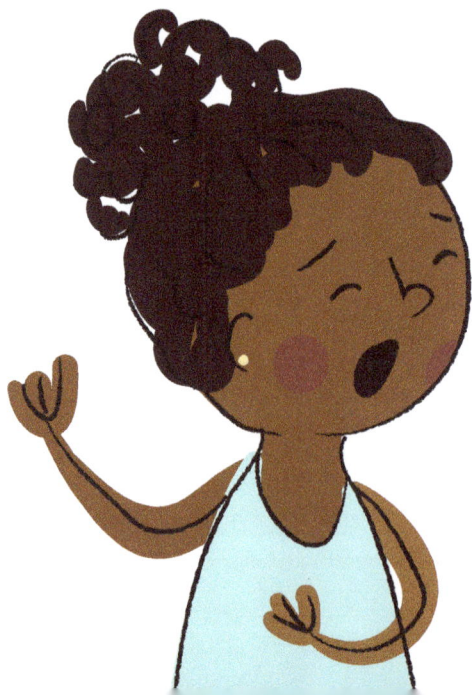

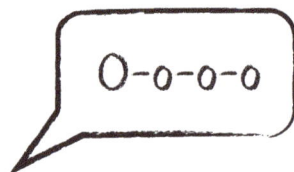

O-o-o-o

LONG VOWELS   SHORT VOWELS

like   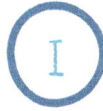   it
virus   is

stay   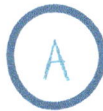   talks
table   what

sneezes   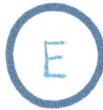   object
disease   gets

crown   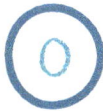   lot
soap   problems

you   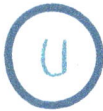   virus
flu   public

HAITI DISCOVERY SERIES

In this series, Petra and Lili discover their country, Haiti, and its rich culture.

You will find level 1, 2, 3 and 4 books to suit the needs of your child or students! Let us know what other parts of Haiti or the Haitian culture you would like Petra and Lili to explore!

TITLES AVAILABLE ON AMAZON AND INGRAM

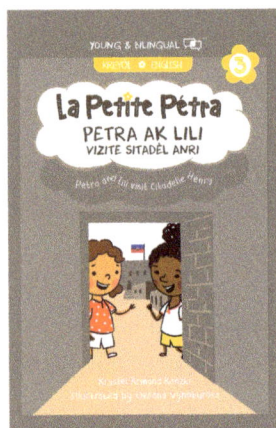

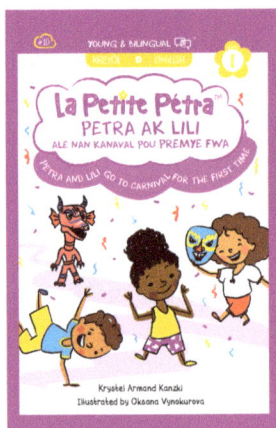

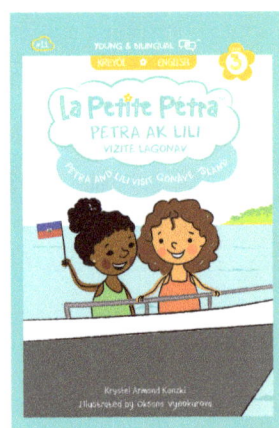

Series also available in Creole/English.

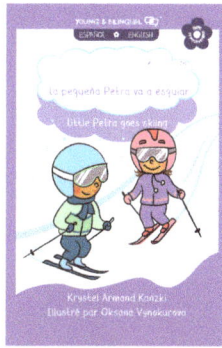

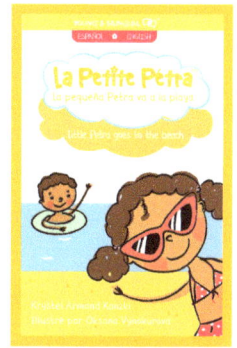

Our bilingual book series also includes books in
Spanish-English
and French-English and some
of our books are available in
Audiobooks to accompany our
young readers! Visit our
website
www.lapetitepetra.com
to view all our titles today!
If your loved ones or
students
benefited from reading this
book, please leave us a
review
on the platform where you
purchased the book and help
us spread the joy!

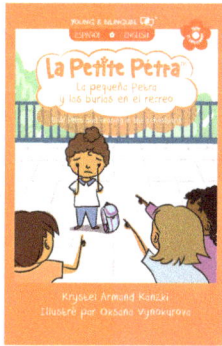

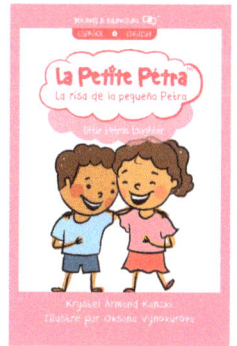

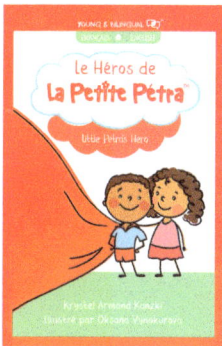

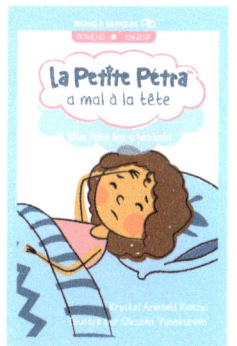

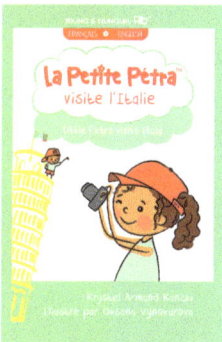

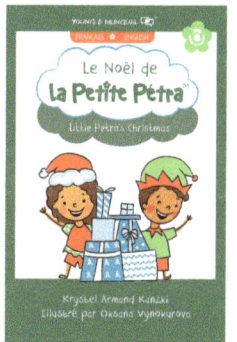

www.ingramcontent.com/pod-product-compliance
Lightning Source LLC
Chambersburg PA
CBHW040830300326
41914CB00085B/2070/J